DIABETES CHEAT CODES 2022:

How to prevent and reverse type 2 diabetes naturally

Dr. Williams Bersus

Table of contents

<h2 align="center">Part one</h2>

- What is Diabetes
- What is blood sugar/Glucose
- Hypoglycemia and Hyperglycemia
- Type of Diabetes, Risk, Factors, and Causes
- How type 2 Diabetes became a plague
- The discrepancy between Type 1 and Type 2 Diabetes
- Effect of Diabetes.

Chapter one

What is Diabetes

The ancient Egyptians spoke of a disease that appears to have been type 1 diabetes more than 3,000 years ago. It included thirst, increased urine, and weight loss. To lessen the symptoms, the authors suggested consuming whole grains in your diet. When your blood glucose, commonly known as blood sugar, is too high, you develop diabetes. Your primary energy source is blood glucose, which is obtained from the food you eat. The pancreas produces the hormone insulin, which facilitates the entry of food-derived glucose into your cells for energy production. Your body occasionally produces insufficient or no insulin, or it uses insulin poorly. After that, glucose remains in your circulation and does not enter your cells.

Having too much glucose in the blood over time may cause health problems. Even though there is no cure for diabetes, you can control it and keep yourself healthy.
Diabetes is sometimes referred to as "borderline diabetes" or "a touch of sugar." These phrases imply that a person doesn't have diabetes or has a less severe condition, however, diabetes always has major consequences. Diabetes is a chronic condition brought on by either insufficient insulin production by the

pancreas or inefficient insulin use by the body. A hormone called insulin controls blood sugar levels. Uncontrolled diabetes often causes hyperglycemia, also known as high blood glucose or raised blood sugar, which over time may seriously harm many different bodily systems, including the neurons and blood vessels.

8.5% of persons who were 18 years of age and older had diabetes in 2014. A total of 1.5 million fatalities were directly related to diabetes in 2019, and 48% of these deaths occurred in those under the age of 70. Diabetes contributed to an additional 460 000 renal disease deaths, and high blood glucose is responsible for 20% of cardiovascular fatalities.

Age-standardized diabetes mortality rates increased by 3% between 2000 and 2019. Diabetes-related death rates rose 13% in lower-middle-income nations.

In contrast, between 2000 and 2019, there was a 22% worldwide decline in the likelihood of dying from any of the four major noncommunicable illnesses (cancer, chronic respiratory diseases, diabetes, or cardiovascular diseases) between the ages of 30 and 70.

Finally, diabetes affects how your body converts food into energy and is a chronic (long-lasting) health issue.

The majority of the food you consume is converted by your body into sugar (glucose), which is then released into your circulation. Your pancreas releases insulin when your blood sugar levels rise. For blood sugar to enter your body's cells and be used as energy, insulin functions like a key.

When you have diabetes, your body either produces insufficient insulin or uses it improperly. Too much blood sugar remains in your circulation when there is insufficient insulin or when cells cease reacting to insulin. That may eventually lead to major health issues including renal disease, eyesight loss, and heart disease.

Although there is currently no treatment for diabetes, decreasing weight, eating well, and exercising may all be very beneficial. Take the prescription medication exactly as directed.

Obtain guidance and information about diabetes self-management.

Schedule and attend medical appointments.

Chapter Two

What is blood sugar/Glucose

Glucose is the Greek word meaning "sweet." This specific kind of sugar, which your body gets from the food you eat, serves as fuel. When blood reaches your cells and travels through your circulation, it is referred to as blood glucose or blood sugar.

Insulin is a hormone that moves glucose from the blood into cells where it may be stored and used as fuel. Diabetics have higher blood glucose levels than healthy individuals. Either they don't have enough insulin to pass it through or their cells don't respond to insulin as they should.

Your kidneys, eyes, and other organs may be harmed by persistently high blood glucose levels.

How Your Body Makes Glucose

It mostly originates from foods high in carbs, such as fruit, bread, and potatoes. Food moves from your mouth to your stomach through your esophagus while you eat. It is reduced to small fragments by acids and enzymes there. This causes the release of glucose.

It enters your intestines to be absorbed there. It then enters your bloodstream from there. Once in circulation, insulin aids in the delivery of glucose to your cells. The primary sugar in your blood is called blood sugar, or glucose. Your body uses it as its primary source of energy, and it originates from the food you consume. All of the cells in your body get glucose from your blood to be used as fuel.

Diabetes is a condition in which you have too high blood sugar levels. Having too much glucose in your blood might have major consequences over time. You could sometimes have issues with too low or too high blood sugar even if you don't have diabetes. Maintaining regular eating, exercise, and medication regimen may assist.

It is crucial to maintain blood sugar levels within your goal range if you have diabetes. Your blood sugar may need to be checked multiple times each day. A blood test known as an A1C will also be performed by your medical professional. It measures your three-month average blood sugar level. You may need to take medications or adhere to a particular diet if your blood sugar level is too high.

Energy and Storage

Your body is built to maintain a consistent blood glucose level. Every few seconds, beta cells in your pancreas check the level of your blood sugar. After eating, the beta cells release insulin into circulation as your blood glucose levels increase. For glucose to enter muscle, fat, and liver cells, insulin works as a key to unlock those cells.

The majority of the cells in your body utilize glucose, lipids, and amino acids (the components of protein) as fuel. However, it serves as your brain's primary source of fuel. It is necessary for information processing by the nerve cells and chemical messengers there. Your brain couldn't function properly without it.

The remaining glucose is stored in tiny bundles called glycogen in the liver and muscles after your body has spent the energy it requires. Your body has enough reserves to last roughly a day.

Your blood glucose level falls a few hours after your last meal. As a result, your pancreas quits producing insulin. A new hormone called glucagon begins to be produced by alpha cells in the pancreas. It instructs the liver to convert glycogen that has been stored into glucose by dissolving it.

From there, it enters your circulation to top up your supply until you can eat again. Additionally, your liver may produce glucose on its own by combining waste materials, amino acids, and lipids.

Blood Glucose and Diabetic Conditions

After eating, your blood sugar level often increases. A few hours later, it falls when insulin transports glucose into your cells. Your blood sugar should be under 100 milligrams per deciliter (mg/dl) between meals. Your fasting blood sugar level is what is meant by this.

Chapter three

Hypoglycemia and Hyperglycemia

Hypoglycemia (Low Blood Sugar)
is a condition when your blood sugar level (glucose) is below the normal range. Your body uses glucose as its primary energy source.

Hypoglycemia and diabetes management often go hand in hand. Low blood sugar may, however, occur in persons without diabetes due to several diseases and other medications, many of which are uncommon. Treating hypoglycemia urgently is necessary. A fasting blood sugar reading of 70 mg/dL, or 3.9 mmol/L, or lower should be seen as a warning sign for hypoglycemia in many individuals. Your figures, however, could be different. Inquire with your doctor.

The goal of treatment is to lower your blood sugar as rapidly as possible, either with a high-sugar meal or beverage or by taking medication. It is necessary to identify and address the source of hypoglycemia for long-term therapy.
Symptoms
Hypoglycemia symptoms and indicators may appear if blood sugar levels go too low and include:

- seeming pale
- Shakiness
- Sweating
- Headache
- Hunger or sickness
- a rapid or erratic pulse
- Fatigue
- irritation or worry
- difficulty paying attention
- Unsteadiness or faintness
- Lips, tongue, or cheek tingling or numbness

Signs and symptoms of hypoglycemia may include:

- Unusual behavior, confusion, or both, such as the inability to carry out daily chores
- Inability to coordinate
- Unsteady speech
- fuzziness or tunnel vision
- nightmares when sleeping
- Extreme hypoglycemia may result in:

- Unresponsiveness (lack of awareness) (loss of consciousness)
- Seizures

When to see a doctor
Immediately seek medical attention if;

You could have signs of hypoglycemia, but you don't have diabetes.

You have diabetes, and despite trying to manage your hypoglycemia by drinking juice or normal (not diet) soft drinks, eating sweets, or taking glucose pills, nothing seems to work.

If you have diabetes or a history of hypoglycemia and you have severe hypoglycemia symptoms or you become unconscious, you should seek immediate medical attention.

Causes

When your blood sugar (glucose) level drops too low for normal body processes to continue, you have hypoglycemia. This may occur for several reasons. Low blood sugar is most often caused by a side effect of diabetic treatments.

Blood sugar regulation

Your body converts food into glucose when you eat. Insulin, a hormone produced by the pancreas, aids in the entry of glucose, the body's primary energy source, into the cells. Insulin enables glucose to enter the cells and provide the energy required by your cells. Your muscles and liver both contain glycogen, which is a sort of extra glucose storage.

You will cease manufacturing insulin when you haven't eaten in many hours and your blood sugar level falls. The pancreatic hormone glucagon instructs your liver to release glucose into your circulation by dissolving the glycogen that has been stored in your body. Until you eat again, this maintains your blood sugar levels within a normal range.

Glucose may also be produced by your body. Your kidneys and liver both play a major role in this process. The body may break down fat reserves and utilize the byproducts of fat breakdown as an alternate fuel during extended fasting.

Possible causes with Diabetes

If you have diabetes, you may not produce insulin (type 1 diabetes) or you may respond to insulin less favorably (type 2 diabetes). As a consequence, blood glucose levels increase and can rise to dangerously high levels. You could use insulin or other blood sugar-lowering drugs to solve this issue.

However, using too much insulin or other diabetic drugs might result in hypoglycemia, which is when your blood sugar level drops too low. In addition, hypoglycemia might happen if you exercise more than normal or if you eat less than usual after taking your daily dosage of diabetic medication. Causes

When your blood sugar (glucose) level drops too low for normal body processes to continue, you have hypoglycemia. This may occur for several reasons. Low blood sugar is most often caused by a side effect of diabetic treatments.

Blood sugar regulation

Your body converts food into glucose when you eat. Insulin, a hormone produced by the pancreas, aids in the entry of glucose, the body's primary energy source, into the cells. Insulin enables glucose to enter the cells and provide the energy required by your cells. Your muscles and liver both contain glycogen, which is a sort of extra glucose storage.

You will cease manufacturing insulin when you haven't eaten in many hours and your blood sugar level falls. The pancreatic hormone glucagon instructs your liver to release glucose into your circulation by dissolving the glycogen that has been stored in your body. Until you eat again, this maintains your blood sugar levels within a normal range.

Glucose may also be produced by your body. Your kidneys and liver both play a major role in this process. The body may break down fat reserves and utilize the byproducts of fat breakdown as an alternate fuel during extended fasting.

Potential causes include diabetes

If you have diabetes, you may not produce insulin (type 1 diabetes) or you may respond to insulin less favorably (type 2 diabetes). As a consequence, blood glucose levels increase and can rise to dangerously high levels. You could use insulin or other blood sugar-lowering drugs to solve this issue.

However, using too much insulin or other diabetic drugs might result in hypoglycemia, which is when your blood sugar level drops too low. In addition, hypoglycemia might happen if you exercise more than normal or if you eat less than usual after taking your daily dosage of diabetic medication.

Possible causes, without Diabetes

Hypoglycemia in people without diabetes is much less common. Causes can include:

- Medications. Accidentally ingesting someone else's oral diabetic medicine might result in hypoglycemia. Other drugs have the potential to induce hypoglycemia, particularly in young patients or those with renal disease. One such is the malaria drug quinine (Qualaquin).
- Excessive alcohol consumption Drinking excessively without eating may prevent the liver from releasing glucose into the circulation from its glycogen reserves. The result may be hypoglycemia; a few serious diseases.

- Hypoglycemia may be brought on by severe infections, renal disease, advanced heart disease, and liver diseases such as severe cirrhosis or hepatitis. Additionally, kidney problems might prevent your body from adequately eliminating drugs. An accumulation of drugs that reduce blood sugar levels, may have an impact on glucose levels.

- Long-term starvation: When you don't eat enough, your body uses up the glycogen reserves it needs to produce glucose, which may lead to hypoglycemia. One condition that may result in hypoglycemia and long-term malnutrition is an eating disorder termed anorexia nervosa.

- Insulin overproduction. You may get hypoglycemia if your pancreas produces too much insulin due to a rare pancreatic tumor called an insulinoma. A surplus of insulin-like molecules may also be produced as a consequence of other cancers. The pancreas' peculiar cells may cause excessive insulin release, which leads to hypoglycemia.

- Hormone deficiencies. Specific diseases of the pituitary and adrenal glands may cause insufficient levels of certain hormones that control glucose synthesis or metabolism. If a child has too little growth hormone, they may have hypoglycemia.

Hypoglycemia after meals

Usually, but not always, hypoglycemia happens after not eating. After certain meals, hypoglycemic symptoms can appear, although it is unclear why.

Reactive hypoglycemia, also known as postprandial hypoglycemia, may happen in patients who have had procedures that alter the stomach's normal function. Although stomach bypass surgery is the procedure most often linked to this, it may also happen to patients who have undergone other procedures.

Complications

Untreated hypoglycemia can lead to:

- Seizure
- Coma
- Death
- Hypoglycemia can also cause:
-
- Dizziness and weakness
- Falls
- Injuries
- Motor vehicle accidents
- Greater risk of dementia in older adults

Hypoglycemia unawareness

Recurrent hypoglycemic episodes may cause hypoglycemia unawareness to gradually emerge over time. The body and brain no longer create low blood sugar warning signs and symptoms like shaking or irregular heartbeats (palpitations). When this happens, the danger of severe, perhaps deadly hypoglycemia increases.

If you have diabetes, recurrent hypoglycemia, and hypoglycemia unawareness, your healthcare provider may adjust your medication, increase your blood sugar level targets, and recommend blood glucose awareness training.

Some individuals who are unaware of their hypoglycemia may utilize a continuous glucose monitor (CGM). It may be too low for your blood sugar, and the device may alert you to it.

Undertreated diabetes

Episodes of low blood sugar are unpleasant and even terrifying if you have diabetes. You may take less insulin out of fear of hypoglycemia to prevent your blood sugar from dropping too low. This may cause diabetes to become unmanageable. Discuss your fears with your healthcare practitioner, and don't alter the dosage of your diabetic medication without first consulting them.

Hyperglycemia (High Blood Sugar) (High Blood Sugar)

Because the body doesn't produce enough insulin, hyperglycemia (high blood glucose) occurs when there is too much sugar in the blood. Hyperglycemia, a sign of diabetes, may lead to vomiting, increased hunger and thirst, a fast pulse, eyesight issues, and other symptoms. Serious health issues might result from untreated hyperglycemia.

What is hyperglycemia?

When the blood sugar level is excessively high, a condition known as hyperglycemia, or high blood glucose, develops. This occurs if your body can't effectively utilize insulin or if there is insufficient insulin in your system (insulin is the hormone that carries glucose into the blood). The disease is often associated with diabetes.

If you have diabetes and your fasting blood sugar is more than 125 mg/dL (milligrams per deciliter), you have hyperglycemia. Fasting is defined as not eating for at least eight hours.

- A person has impaired glucose tolerance, or pre-diabetes, with a fasting blood glucose of 100 mg/dL to 125 mg/dL.
- A person has hyperglycemia if their blood glucose is greater than 180 mg/dL one to two hours after eating.

Your neurons, blood vessels, tissues, and organs might be harmed if hyperglycemia is left untreated for an extended length of time. Your risk of heart attack and stroke may rise if your blood vessels are damaged, and kidney damage, eye damage, and non-healing wounds can all result from nerve damage as well.

What are risk factors for hyperglycemia?
Major risk factors for hyperglycemia are:

- You have a family history of type 2 diabetes.
- You are African American, Native American, Hispanic or Asian American.
- You are overweight.
- You have high blood pressure or cholesterol.
- You have polycystic ovarian syndrome (PCOS).
- You have a history of gestational diabetes.

What causes hyperglycemia in people with diabetes

- The dose of insulin or oral diabetes medication that you are taking is not the most helpful dose for your needs.
- Your body isn't using your natural insulin effectively (type 2 diabetes).
- The amount of carbohydrates you are eating or drinking is not balanced with the amount of insulin your body is able to make or the amount of insulin you inject.
- You are less active than usual.

- Physical stress (from illness, a cold, the flu, an infection, etc.) is affecting you.
- Emotional stress (from family conflicts, emotional problems, school or work stresses, etc.) is affecting you.
- You are taking steroids for another condition.
- The dawn phenomenon (a surge of hormones the body produces every morning around 4 am to 5 a.m.) is affecting you.

Other possible causes

- Endocrine conditions, such as Cushing syndrome, that cause insulin resistance.
- Pancreatic diseases such as pancreatitis, pancreatic cancer and cystic fibrosis.
- Certain medications (such as diuretics and steroids).
- Gestational diabetes, which happens in 4% of pregnancies, and is due to decreased insulin sensitivity.
- Surgery or trauma

What are the symptoms of hyperglycemia?

Knowing the early warning signals of hyperglycemia is crucial if you have type 1 diabetes. In persons with type 1 diabetes, uncontrolled hyperglycemia may progress to ketoacidosis, when harmful acids called ketones accumulate in the blood. This emergency circumstance has the potential to cause death or a coma.

Early symptoms of hyperglycemia include:

- High blood sugar.
- Increased thirst and/or hunger.
- Blurred vision.
- Frequent urination (peeing).
- Headache.

Additional symptoms include:

- Fatigue (feeling weak, tired).
- Weight loss.
- Vaginal and skin infections.
- Slow-healing cuts and sores.

Symptoms of ketoacidosis are:

- Vomiting.
- Dehydration.
- Unusual fruity smell on the breath.
- Deep labored breathing or hyperventilation.
- Rapid heartbeat.
- Confusion and disorientation.
- Coma.

How can I treat and manage hyperglycemia?

Both type 1 and type 2 diabetics may control hyperglycemia by maintaining a nutritious diet, getting enough exercise, and reducing stress. Additionally, patients with type 1 diabetes must use insulin to control their hyperglycemia, but those with type 2 diabetes may first need to use oral medicines before switching to insulin.

Call your healthcare practitioner if you don't have diabetes but exhibit any hyperglycemia-related symptoms. You can control your hyperglycemia by working together.

How do I prevent hyperglycemia?

- Exercise to help lower blood sugar. Work with your healthcare provider to make a daily activity plan.
- Follow your meal plan if you have one. Learn how carbohydrates impact your blood sugar, and work with your diabetes care team to find the best meal plan for you.
- Maintain a healthy weight.
- Don't smoke.
- Limit drinking alcohol. Alcohol can raise blood sugar levels, but can also cause dangerously low blood sugar levels. Work with your provider to determine how much is safe to drink.

Chapter Four

Type of Diabetes, Risk, Factors, and Causes.

The types of diabetes are:

Type 1 diabetes:

An autoimmune illness of this kind causes the body to fight itself. In this situation, your pancreas' insulin-producing cells are killed. Type 1 diabetes affects up to 10% of patients with the disease. Typically, children and young adults get the diagnosis (but can develop at any age). Diabetes used to be more often recognized as "juvenile" diabetes. Those who have Type 1 diabetes must take insulin daily. It is also known as insulin-dependent diabetes for this reason.

Type 2 diabetes:

With this kind of, either your body doesn't produce enough insulin or your cells don't react to the insulin as they should. The most typical kind of diabetes is this one. Up to 95% of those who have diabetes are Type 2 patients. People in their middle years and older tend to develop it. Insulin-resistant diabetes and adult-onset diabetes are two more names for Type 2. "Having a bit of sugar" is what your parents or grandparents could have described it as.

Prediabetes:

The stage of diabetes preceding Kind 2 is this type. Your blood glucose levels are above average but not high enough to get a Type 2 diabetes diagnosis.
Gestational diabetes: This kind appears in certain pregnant women. After pregnancy, gestational diabetes often disappears. However, if you have gestational diabetes, you are more likely to eventually acquire Type 2 diabetes.
Diabetes may occur in less prevalent forms like:

Monogenic diabetes syndromes: Up to 4% of cases of diabetes are caused by these uncommon hereditary types of the disease. Examples include young-onset diabetes with maturity and neonatal diabetes.
Diabetes associated with cystic fibrosis: This is a kind of diabetes that only affects those who have this condition.
Diabetes brought on by drugs or chemicals: Symptoms of this kind include organ transplantation, HIV/AIDS therapy, and the usage of glucocorticoids.
Your kidneys create a lot of pee when you have diabetes insipidus, a unique unusual illness.

How common is diabetes?

In the United States, 34.2 million individuals of all ages, or nearly 1 in 10, have diabetes. A little less than 3% of all individuals in the United States, or around 7.3 million people, are ignorant that they have diabetes. As individuals become older, more people are getting diabetes diagnoses. About 1 in 4 persons (about 26% of those over 65) have diabetes.

Who gets diabetes? What are the risk factors?

Factors that increase your risk differ depending on the type of diabetes you ultimately develop.

Risk factors for Type 1 diabetes include:

having a parent or sibling who has type 1 diabetes.
a pancreatic injury (such as by infection, tumor, surgery, or accident).
autoantibodies, or antibodies that erroneously target the tissues or organs of your own body, are present.
physical adversity (such as surgery or illness).
exposure to virus-based diseases
Prediabetes and Type 2 diabetes are both at risk for:

family history of Type 2 diabetes or prediabetes (parent or sibling).
being a person of African, Hispanic, Native American, Asian, or Pacific Islander descent.
being overweight or obese.
blood pressure being high.
a high triglyceride level and low HDL cholesterol (the "good" cholesterol).
being inactive physically.

45 years of age or more.
gestational diabetes or having a baby that weighs more than nine pounds.
a polycystic ovary syndrome patient.
a history of cardiovascular disease or stroke.
cigarette smoking
Pregnancy-related diabetes risk factors include:
Family history (parent or sibling) of prediabetes or Type 2 diabetes.
Being African-American, Hispanic, Native American or Asian-American.
Having been overweight/obesity before your pregnancy.
Being over 25 years of age.

SYMPTOMS AND CAUSES

What causes diabetes?

No of the kind, having too much glucose flowing in your circulation is what causes diabetes. However, depending on the kind of diabetes you have, there are several causes for elevated blood glucose levels.

Type 1 diabetes has immune system-related causes. Your body assaults and kills the cells in your pancreas that make insulin. Glucose builds up in your circulation without insulin, which allows glucose to enter your cells. Some patients may also be affected by their genes. A virus may also set off an immune system response.

Cause of Type 2 diabetes and prediabetes:

The cells in your body prevent insulin from working as it should permit glucose to enter the cells. The cells in your body are no longer susceptible to insulin. To produce enough insulin to overcome this resistance, your pancreas cannot keep up. The amount of glucose in your blood increases.

Gestational diabetes: While you are pregnant, the placenta releases hormones that make your body's cells more resistant to the effects of insulin. Insufficient insulin is produced by your pancreas to overcome this resistance. There is still too much glucose in your blood.

What are the symptoms of diabetes?
Symptoms of diabetes include:

Increased thirst.
Weak, tired feeling.
Blurred vision.
Numbness or tingling in the hands or feet.
Slow-healing sores or cuts.
Unplanned weight loss.
Frequent urination.
Frequent unexplained infections.
Dry mouth.
Other symptoms

Frequently occurring yeast infections or urinary tract infections in women, as well as dry, itchy skin.
Erectile dysfunction diminished muscular strength and decreased sex desire in males.

Diabetes type 1 symptoms The onset of symptoms may take just a few weeks or months. The first signs usually appear in childhood, adolescence, or early adulthood. Yeast infections or urinary tract infections, as well as nausea, vomiting, or stomach aches, are other symptoms.

Type 2 diabetes and prediabetes symptoms: Given that they appear gradually over many years, you could not have any symptoms at all or fail to recognize them. Although prediabetes and Type 2 diabetes are becoming more prevalent across all age groups, symptoms often start to appear when a person is an adult.

Gestational diabetes:

Typically, you won't feel any symptoms. Between 24 and 28 weeks of your pregnancy, your obstetrician will do a gestational diabetes screening on you.

What are the complications of diabetes?
Your body's tissues and organs may sustain severe harm if your blood glucose level is high for an extended length of time. Over time, certain issues may pose a danger to life.

Complications include:

Cardiovascular issues including coronary artery disease, chest pain, heart attack, stroke, high blood pressure,

high cholesterol, atherosclerosis (narrowing of the arteries).
Nerve damage (neuropathy) that causes numbing and tingling that starts at toes or fingers then spreads.
Kidney damage (nephropathy) that can lead to kidney failure or the need for dialysis or transplant.
Eye damage (retinopathy) that can lead to blindness; cataracts, glaucoma.
Foot damage including nerve damage, poor blood flow and poor healing of cuts and sores.
Skin infections.
Erectile dysfunction.
Hearing loss.
Depression.
Dementia.
Dental problems.
Complications of gestational diabetes:

In the mother: Preeclampsia (high blood pressure, excess protein in urine, leg/feet swelling), risk of gestational diabetes during future pregnancies and risk of diabetes later in life.

In the newborn: Higher-than-normal birth weight, low blood sugar (hypoglycemia), higher risk of developing Type 2 diabetes over time and death shortly after birth.

Gestational diabetes tests: If you are pregnant, there are two blood glucose tests. In a glucose challenge test, you consume a sweet beverage, after which your blood sugar level is measured an hour later. Before this exam, you don't need to fast. An oral glucose tolerance test will come next if this test reveals a higher than-usual amount of glucose (above 140 ml/dL) (as described above).

Type 1 diabetes: Blood and urine samples will be taken, and examined if your doctor suspects Type 1 diabetes. Checks are made for autoantibodies in the blood (an autoimmune sign that your body is attacking itself). The presence of ketones in the urine is examined (a sign your body is burning fat as its energy supply). These symptoms are a marker of Type 1 diabetes.

Who should be tested for diabetes?
You should be checked if you have diabetes or any of its risk factors. Diabetes may be managed and problems can be mitigated or avoided the sooner they are discovered. If a blood test reveals you have prediabetes, you may work with your healthcare provider to adopt lifestyle changes (such as losing weight, exercising, and eating a nutritious diet) to stop or postpone the onset of Type 2 diabetes.

Additional specific testing advice based on risk factors:

Testing for Type 1 diabetes: Children and young adults with a family history of diabetes should be tested. Less often, Type 1 diabetes may also strike elderly persons. Therefore, it's crucial to examine people who visit the hospital and are discovered to be suffering from diabetes-related ketoacidosis. A potentially fatal complication that may happen to someone with Type 1 diabetes is ketoacidosis.

Testing for type 2 diabetes: Test older individuals (over the age of 45), people between the ages of 19 and 44 who are overweight or obese and have one or more risk factors, pregnant women, and kids (aged 10 to 18) who are overweight or obese and have at least two risk factors for type 2 diabetes.

Gestational diabetes: All pregnant women with diabetes should be tested. Between weeks 24 and 28, provide a pregnancy test to all pregnant women. Your obstetrician may test you early if you have additional gestational diabetes risk factors.

Before a meal: between 80 and 130 mg/dL.

About two hours after the start of a meal: less than 180 mg/dL.

What happens if my blood glucose level is low?

Having a blood glucose level that is lower than the normal range (usually below 70 mg/dL) is called hypoglycemia. This is a sign that your body gives out that you need sugar.

Symptoms you might experience if you have hypoglycemia include:

Weakness or shaking.
Moist skin, sweating.
Fast heartbeat.
Dizziness.

Sudden hunger.
Confusion.
Pale skin.
Numbness in mouth or tongue.
Irritability, nervousness.
Unsteadiness.
Nightmares, bad dreams, restless sleep.
Blurred vision.
Headaches, seizures.
You might pass out if your hypoglycemia is not managed.

Chapter Five

How type 2 Diabetes became a plague

Diabetes, more especially type 2 diabetes, is a wholly contemporary disease that is haunting developed-world consumers, spreading via our crammed shopping carts and plates, and finding root in our expanding waistlines. In the eldritch peloton of the Riders of the Apocalypse, type-2 is easy to identify since he is the overweight kid at the rear.

Not because of any inherent sexism, but rather because males are naturally more vulnerable to the sickness, I employ the third person masculine here. Men are more likely to acquire the condition with lower body mass indices, maybe because our fat tends to accumulate around the midsection while women's fat is spread more equally throughout the body. However, we know very little about diabetes and its causes. Asking your pals about it will likely get an unreliable answer along the lines of, "It has something to do with sugar, isn't it?" As if avoiding banoffee pie would make them invulnerable.

I can provide you with a few concrete statistics that show how the sickness is slowly spreading around the UK, but one stands out to me as being speculative. Although 4.5 million individuals have received a diagnosis, it is believed that another 630,000 people have the illness unknowingly. According to Libby Dowling, clinical advisor at Diabetes UK, type-2 diabetes doesn't initially cause significant changes in how you feel. Before it is discovered, some people have been known to live with it for up to 10 years. If it's not impacting your health, is this still a problem? It is a big one, indeed. Even when diabetes is properly controlled, certain of your main organs might gradually lose function over time. Unchecked, it may cause damage. Hospital doctor and writer Max Pemberton recently stated he'd prefer to be diagnosed as HIV positive than diabetic in a usual whip-smart and controversial post. For the former, improvements in antiretroviral medications have transformed the effective death sentence of the 1980s and 1990s into a treatable illness. Although the virus hasn't been eradicated, it has been stopped. Diabetes, however, is still developing. According to Pemberton, "the risk of stroke among newly treated type-2 diabetes is more than double that of the general population." "Diabetics increase the risk of cardiovascular disease by four times. In 20 to 30% of diabetics, damage to the renal filtering system results in kidney failure and the need for dialysis. Blindness is often brought on by damage to the delicate veins in the eyes, and foot sores and ulcers, which require amputating the foot and leg, are sometimes brought on by damage to nerves.

Diabetes has grown unnoticed in comparison to the ominous public health warnings that formerly followed the emergence of HIV, acting as a John Hurt-voiced Götterdämmerung for the liberal culture. It's gotten so typical that it's almost tempting to think of it as an inevitable aspect of getting older. According to Dowling, "since it impacts so many people, it's not treated as seriously as it ought to be." Not only by the patients but also by the caregivers.

But Pemberton bluntly portrayed the bleak reality. Access to the most recent treatments means that for patients residing in the industrialized world, "HIV no longer affects your life expectancy, whereas type-2 diabetes often reduces it by 10 years."

"We're dying of ignorance in slow motion. Or, maybe more concerning, of complacency.

If you're a male, at least, there are two distinct types of diabetes. Since type-1 is an autoimmune illness that often manifests in childhood, there isn't much you can do about it. At this point, the pancreas quits manufacturing the insulin required for the body to use blood sugar as fuel. As a consequence, the body will start using alternative energy sources, such as fat cells, which may cause a toxic overload.

Type-2 diabetes, often known as adult-onset diabetes, accounts for 90% of cases. The pancreas is still producing some insulin in this situation, but not enough or of high enough quality. Blood that is high in glucose rushes through the body as a consequence, harming both large blood arteries like those that link with the heart, and smaller vessels like those that travel to the kidneys and the eyes. According to Dowling, "it roughens the interior of them, producing clotting and harming internal organs."

Your Sugar Fix

How can you avoid it? Age (after 40, or 25 if you're of South Asian descent), family history, and weight are the three main risk factors. You can't do much about the first two, but you can put the pie down. According to Dowling, being overweight causes the body to become significantly more resistant to insulin. The pancreas will begin to flood the body with insulin until it stops generating anymore, for reasons we do not fully understand. At this point, you'll need to start injecting insulin, but if you discover the condition early enough, you may manage it without medication by engaging in regular exercise and eating a balanced diet.

Diabetes UK is cautiously enthusiastic about research into low-calorie diets even though a cure for diabetes is still elusive. Eight weeks into a 600-calorie diet, volunteers saw their blood sugar levels fall below the diabetic threshold. Outside of a scientific study, it is highly difficult and perhaps harmful to follow the regimen. However, it does pave the way for further discoveries. According to Dowling, "Type-2 tends to go into remission; it's too soon to declare it's been healed."

However, we have continued to finance this very promising study through 2018.

Exercise, eat well, and avoid using the spare tire in the meantime. Simple but necessary procedures to avoid the needle and the harm done.

Chapter Six

The discrepancy between Type 1 and Type 2 Diabetes

Type 1 diabetes is a hereditary illness that often manifests in childhood, but type 2 diabetes is mostly connected to lifestyle choices and develops over time. Your immune system attacks and kills the insulin-producing cells in your pancreas when you have type 1 diabetes.
There are several distinctions between type 1 and type 2 diabetes, even though they share certain characteristics. such as their origins, the people they touch, and management strategies.

To begin with, type 1 affects 8% of all diabetics. while 90% of people with diabetes are type 2.

Type 1 and type 2 diabetes are often mistaken. This might need you to explain that there are several reasons and that what works for one kind doesn't work for the other.

The most important thing to keep in mind is that both are equally serious. Whether you have type 1 or type 2 diabetes, having high blood glucose (or sugar) levels may cause major health consequences. Therefore, if you have either illness, you must manage it properly.

Type 1 and type 2 differences

Below is a guide to some of the main differences between type 1 and type 2.

	Type 1	Type 2
What's happening?	Your body attacks the cells in your pancreas which means it cannot make any insulin.	Your body is unable to make enough insulin or the insulin you do make doesn't work properly.
Risk factors	We don't currently know what causes type 1 diabetes.	We know some things can put you at risk of having type 2 like weight and ethnicity.
Symptoms	We know some things can put you at risk of having type 2 like weight and ethnicity	Type 2 symptoms can be easier to miss because they appear more slowly.

Management	Type 1 is managed by taking insulin to control your blood sugar.	You can manage type 2 diabetes in more ways than type 1. These include through medication, exercise and diet. People with type 2 can also be prescribed insulin.
Cure factors	Currently there is no cure for type 1 but research continues.	Type 2 cannot be cured but there is evidence to say in many cases it can be prevented and put into remission.

What happens when you have type 1 and type 2 diabetes?

Diabetes, whether type 1 or type 2, is characterized by an excess of glucose (a form of sugar) in the blood. This is true for both kinds. However, how this occurs varies among them.

Type 1 diabetes is an indication of an autoimmune disorder. This indicates that your body has attacked and killed the cells responsible for producing the hormone insulin. So you can no longer produce insulin.

We all need insulin because it aids in transporting glucose from the blood into the cells of our bodies. After that, we utilize this glucose as fuel. Your blood glucose level becomes too high if you don't have insulin. Diabetes type 2 is distinct. If you have type 2, either your body doesn't produce enough insulin or your insulin is ineffective. Insulin resistance is the term for this. Similar to type 1, this denotes a very high blood glucose level.

Are there different risk factors for type 1 and type 2?

We don't know exactly what causes type 1 or type 2 diabetes, but we do know the different risk factors. so we know why you might be likely to get one type over the other. Even though we know this, it's good to remember these aren't set in stone.

Type 1

A big difference between the two is that type 1 isn't affected by your lifestyle. Or your weight. That means you can't affect your risk of developing type 1 by lifestyle changes.

People up to the age of 40 are more likely to be diagnosed with it, especially children. In fact, most children with diabetes have type 1. But, although it's less common, people over 40 can also be diagnosed with it.

Type 2

It's different for type 2 diabetes. We know some things put you at more risk:

- your family history
- ethnic background
- age
- if you're overweight or obese

We also know that there are things you can do to reduce your risk of developing type 2 diabetes. Things like eating healthily, being active and maintaining a healthy weight can help you to prevent type 2.

You're also more likely to get type 2 if you're over 40. Or if you're South Asian, if you're over 25. But type 2 is also becoming more common in younger people. More and more children and young people get diagnosed with type 2 in the UK each year.

Symptoms of type 1 and type 2

Type 1 and type 2 diabetes share common symptoms. They are:

- going to the toilet a lot, especially at night
- being really thirsty
- feeling more tired than usual
- losing weight without trying to
- genital itching or thrush
- cuts and wounds take longer to heal
- blurred vision.

But where type 1 and type 2 diabetes are different in symptom is how they appear. Type 1 can often appear quite quickly. That makes them harder to ignore. This is important because symptoms that are ignored can lead to diabetic ketoacidosis (DKA).

However, type 2 diabetes can be easier to miss. This is because it develops more slowly, especially in the early stages. That makes it harder to spot the symptoms. That is why it is important to know your risk of developing type 2 diabetes. Some people have diabetes and don't know it. They can have it for up to 10 years without knowing.

The emotional impact of type 1 and type 2 diabetes

Sometimes having diabetes, whether type 1 or type 2, might seem overwhelming.

Although the two forms vary, anybody might experience depression or anxiety as a result of having diabetes.

Understanding that a long-term ailment may have an emotional effect regardless of how it was brought on or how you manage it is crucial.

Remember that you are not alone if you are having trouble managing your diabetes.

You have access to a multitude of resources, including our hotline. There, you may discuss your feelings with one of our highly qualified counselors. Additionally, you may communicate with folks having comparable experiences on our forum. It simply takes discovering what works for you out of all the things you can do to assist yourself.

It might be difficult to describe the variations between type 1 and type 2.

Both kinds struggle with uncertainty over the condition's origins and available treatments. If you have type 1 diabetes or the more prevalent type 2, this will be a little bit different. Something is not always understood just because it is more widespread.

And even if correcting people all the time drains your emotions, you should be aware that you're not the only one. Regardless of the kind, many individuals with diabetes face the same issues and challenges. In the forum and at neighborhood groups, you may get in touch with them to provide or receive help.

Chapter Seven

Effect of Diabetes

The first thing likely comes to mind when you hear the phrase "diabetes" is probably elevated blood sugar.

An often underappreciated aspect of your health is blood sugar. Diabetes may result from a long-term imbalance that is out of balance.

Diabetic issues

Your body's capacity to make or utilize insulin, a hormone that enables your body to convert glucose (sugar) into energy, is referred to as your body's capacity.

Here are some signs of diabetes that you could experience in your body.

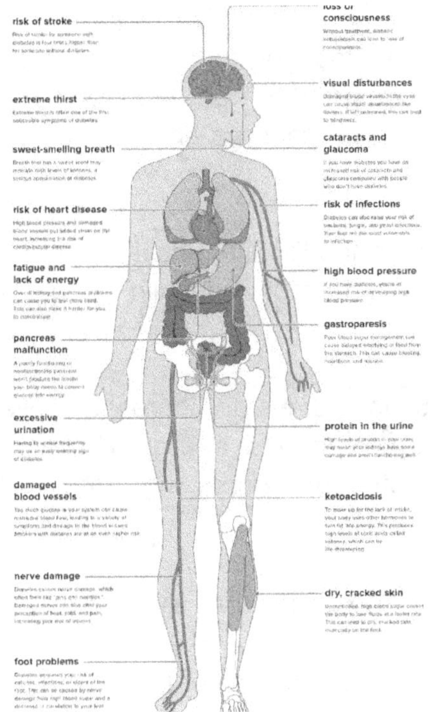

Diabetes can be effectively managed when diagnosed early. However, when left untreated, it can lead to potential complications that include:

- heart disease
- stroke
- kidney damage
- nerve damage

Usually, after eating or drinking, your body will digest the sugars in the meal and utilize them to fuel your cells.

Your pancreas must create the hormone insulin to do this. The process of removing sugar from the blood and delivering it to the cells for utilization as energy is made easier by insulin.

Your pancreas either generates too little insulin or none at all if you have diabetes. Effective insulin usage is impossible.

This permits blood glucose levels to increase while depriving the rest of your cells of vital energy. This may result in a broad range of issues impacting almost all major bodily systems.

Endocrine, excretory, and digestive systems

Other hormones are utilized to convert fat into energy if your pancreas produces little or no insulin or if your body is unable to utilize it. Due to the high quantities of hazardous compounds that may be produced, such as acids and ketone bodies, diabetic ketoacidosis may result. Diabetes has a dangerous consequence called diabetic ketoacidosis. These signs include:

- extreme thirst
- excessive urination
- fatigue

Your breath may smell good because your blood levels of ketones have risen. High blood sugar levels and a lot of ketones in your urine may both be signs of diabetic ketoacidosis. If this disease is not addressed, it might result in death or possibly unconsciousness.

Type 2 diabetes may result in diabetic hyperglycemic hyperosmolar syndrome (HHS). High blood glucose levels are involved, but there are no ketones.

With this disease, dehydration may occur.
Even losing consciousness is possible.
People with untreated diabetes or those who have had trouble managing their diabetes are more likely to develop HHS.
Infection, a stroke, or a heart attack are other potential causes.

Gastroparesis may be brought on by high blood sugar levels.
Your stomach will find it difficult to empty at this time.
The blood sugar levels may increase as a result of this delay.
You could therefore experience:

- Nausea
- Vomiting
- Bloating
- Heartburn

PART TWO

- Early signs, Remedy
- How to effectively treat type 2 Diabetes
- Healthy meals for people with Diabetes

Chapter Eight

Early signs Diabetes, Symptoms of Diabetes 1 and Type 2 Diabetes, Gestational Diabetes, Hypoglycemia, Hyperglycemia and Remedy

Both types of diabetes have some of the same telltale warning signs.

> Hunger and exhaustion Your body transforms the food you consume into glucose, which is then used as energy by your cells. But for your cells to absorb glucose, they require insulin. You won't have any or enough energy if your cells reject the insulin your body produces or if your body doesn't produce any insulin at all. You may get more fatigued and hungry than normal as a result.

- being thirsty and urinating more often The typical individual typically has to urinate four to seven times in 24 hours, but diabetics may urinate far more often. Why? Normally, when glucose goes through your kidneys, your body reabsorbs it. However, when diabetes raises blood sugar levels, your kidneys may not be able to filter everything back into your body. The body produces more pee as a result, which requires fluids. As a consequence, you'll need to visit more often. You could urinate more as well. You may get quite thirsty as a result of your frequent urination. You'll urinate more if you consume more alcohol.

- Itchy skin and a dry mouth. There is less moisture available for other things since your body is utilizing fluids to urinate. Your mouth could feel dry and you might get dehydrated. Your skin may itch if it is dry.
- distorted vision Your eyes' lenses might enlarge due to changes in your body's fluid levels. They alter the form and lose concentration.

Symptoms of Type 2 Diabetes

These tend to show up after your glucose has been high for a long time.

- Yeast infections. Both men and women with diabetes can get these. Yeast feeds on glucose, so having plenty around makes it thrive. Infections can grow in any warm, moist fold of skin, including:
  - Between fingers and toes
  - Under breasts
  - In or around sex organs

- slow-healing cuts or sores. High blood sugar levels over time can impair your blood flow and harm your nerves, making it difficult for your body to heal wounds.
- Pain or numbness in your feet or legs. This is another result of nerve damage.

Symptoms of Type 1 Diabetes

You might notice:

- Unexpected weight loss. Your body will begin burning muscle and fat for energy if it is unable to get it from diet. Even when your eating habits haven't altered, you could still lose weight. Find out which foods contain a lot of trans fatty acids.b
- Nausea and vomiting. Your body produces ketones when it switches to fat burning. These may accumulate in your blood to risky levels, a condition known as diabetic ketoacidosis that may be life-threatening. Your stomach may feel ill after consuming ketones.

Symptoms of Gestational Diabetes

Pregnancy-related high blood sugar often has no symptoms. You can have a little increase in thirst or frequent urination.

Warning Signs of Diabetes Complications

- Signs of type 2 diabetes' complications may include:

- Slow-healing sores or cuts
- Itchy skin (usually around the vaginal or groin area)
- Frequent yeast infections
- Recent weight gain
- Velvety, dark skin changes of the neck, armpit, and groin, called acanthosis nigricans
- Numbness and tingling of the hands and feet
- Decreased vision
- Impotence or erectile dysfunction (ED

Hypoglycemia

When the amount of sugar or glucose in your blood falls too low for the body to use as fuel, you experience hypoglycemia, also known as low blood sugar. You may experience:

- Shaky
- Nervous or anxious
- Sweaty, chilly, or clammy
- Cranky or impatient
- Confused
- Lightheaded or dizzy
- Hungry
- Sleepy

- Weak
- Tingly or numb in your lips, tongue, or cheeks

You might notice:

- Fast heartbeat
- Pale skin
- Blurred vision
- Headache
- Nightmares or crying when you sleep
- Coordination problems
- Seizures

Hyperglycemia

Hyperglycemia, or high blood sugar, causes many of the warning signs of diabetes listed above, including:

- Heavy thirst
- Blurry vision
- Peeing a lot
- More hunger
- Numb or tingling feet
- Fatigue
- Sugar in your urine
- Weight loss
- Vaginal and skin infections
- Slow-healing cuts and sores
- Blood glucose over 180 milligrams per deciliter (mg/dl)

Remedy

The diabetes capital of the globe is allegedly India. With roughly 50 million Indians suffering from diabetes, the nation faces significant obstacles. Let's first discuss what diabetes is. Diabetes is a condition marked by increased blood sugar levels. A person develops diabetes for two main reasons: first, when their body stops making insulin, and second when their body does not react to the insulin that is created by their body. The body converts insulin into energy, which is then sent to the cells. Type I diabetes and Type II diabetes are the two kinds of disease. Let's learn a bit more about them:

Type I diabetes

Juvenile diabetes is another name for type I diabetes, which often affects persons under the age of 20. In this kind, the body loses some or all of its ability to manufacture insulin. Diabetes type I is an autoimmune condition. This occurs when the pancreas, which is where insulin is created, is attacked by the immune system, rendering the pancreas ineffective or unable to produce insulin. Only healthy lifestyle modifications may prevent type I diabetes; it cannot be cured.

Type II diabetes

In India, Type II diabetes is more prevalent than Type I diabetes. Persons over 40 are more likely than younger people to develop type II diabetes. Insulin resistance is the underlying cause of this form of diabetes. In this instance, the body is unable to adequately use the insulin that the pancreas generates. Type II diabetes may be caused by a variety of factors. Being overweight, having high blood pressure, eating poorly, being too stressed, having hormone imbalances, using certain drugs, and living a sedentary lifestyle are a few of the causes. Nevertheless, type II diabetes is reversible.

Let's us know some natural ways by which we can treat diabetes at home:

What not to eat:

Certain meals might have a detrimental effect on your diabetes. Therefore, the first thing you should do is stop eating these things.

Refined sugar - We all understand that sugar is harmful to diabetics unless it is consumed in its most natural form. When ingested, refined sugar causes a sharp rise in blood sugar. Even natural sugars like honey may produce a sharp rise in blood sugar levels. So, if you have diabetes, it is best to avoid refined sugar at all costs.

Whole grains - Gluten-containing grains should be avoided. Diabetes and gluten are linked because eating gluten may result in a leaky gut, which can induce inflammation and, eventually, autoimmune illnesses.

Alcohol - Diabetes and alcohol use are intimately associated. Alcohol destroys your pancreas, which makes insulin, in addition to harming your liver. Two to three glasses of strong alcohol per day are associated with diabetes. Because it contains a lot of carbs, beer should be avoided in particular.

Cow's milk - Cow milk may stimulate the immune system, which can cause inflammation, much as whole grains do. Sheep and goat milk is not toxic; in fact, it aids in blood sugar regulation. But if you have diabetes, drinking regular cow milk might be harmful to you.

GMO foods - GMO foods have the potential to worsen liver and renal conditions as well as increase diabetes. Choose items that are marked as GMO-free.

What to eat and do

Cinnamon

A bioactive component found in cinnamon has the potential to combat and prevent diabetes. It is well known that cinnamon increases insulin action, which lowers blood sugar levels. Like too much of anything is harmful, too much cinnamon may raise the risk of liver damage since it contains a substance called coumarin. It is safer to own genuine cinnamon rather than Cassia cinnamon, which is the kind sold in stores.

How to consume cinnamon

- Mix half or one teaspoon of grounded cinnamon with warm water and have it once daily.
- Boil raw cinnamon in 2 glasses of water. Let it cool for 30 minutes and have it daily.

Aloe vera

Aloe vera is widely available in Indian homes. Even though it has a bitter flavor, mixing it with buttermilk improves the flavor. Aloe vera is often used in cosmetic products, but since it has anti-inflammatory characteristics, it may also treat wounds. It has anti-inflammatory qualities and is thought to regulate blood sugar levels.

Jamun

Blood sugar levels may be lowered with the use of Jamun and its leaves. It is stated that consuming 100 grams of Jamun per day would significantly enhance your blood sugar levels.

Vitamin C

Vitamin C benefits diabetes as well as the skin. According to recent research, taking 600 mg of vitamin C daily may considerably lower blood sugar levels. People with long-term diabetes should regularly eat foods high in vitamin C. Oranges, tomatoes, amla, and blueberries are a few examples of foods high in vitamin C.

Exercise

One of the main reasons behind type II diabetes is being overweight. Any kind of physical activity, be it yoga, Zumba, aerobics, gymming, playing sports can significantly improve blood sugar level by maintaining your weight. Not only this, walking every day can help to reduce the blood sugar level tremendously.

3 ways to reduce your risk of diabetes

Choose water as your primary beverage

By choosing water as your primary beverage, you may stay away from other drinks that are full of sugar and preservatives.
Adults with type 2 diabetes and latent autoimmune diabetes are more likely to consume sugary drinks..

Lose weight if you are overweight

Although type 2 diabetes does not always occur in overweight or obese adults, it does in the majority of cases. The risk of developing diabetes is markedly increased by excess visceral fat, which encourages inflammation and insulin resistance.

Your chance of developing type 2 diabetes is reduced by even 10% weight loss. The general guideline is that you will get more advantages as you lose more.

Quit smoking

Numerous major medical issues have been associated with smoking. Additionally, studies have indicated that smoking and passive smoking increase the risk of type 2 diabetes.
Smoking raises diabetes risk by 44%, and the risk rises to 61% for those who smoke more than 20 cigarettes each day.

Chapter Nine

How to effectively treat type 2 Diabetes

Diagnosis

To diagnose type 2 diabetes, the glycated hemoglobin (A1C) test is often utilized. This blood test measures your average blood sugar level during the past two to three months. The findings are interpreted as follows:

- Below 5.7% is normal.
- 5.7% to 6.4% is diagnosed as prediabetes.
- 6.5% or higher on two separate tests indicates diabetes.

If the A1C test isn't available or if you have certain circumstances that interfere with an A1C test, your doctor may use the following tests to diagnose diabetes:

Random blood sugar test. Millimoles of sugar per liter (mmol/L) of blood or milligrams of sugar per deciliter (mg/dL) is used to express blood sugar levels. No matter when you last ate, a level of 200 mg/dL (11.1 mmol/L) or above indicates diabetes, particularly if you also exhibit symptoms of diabetes like severe thirst and frequent urination.

Fasting blood sugar test. A blood sample is taken after an overnight fast. Results are interpreted as follows:

- Less than 100 mg/dL (5.6 mmol/L) is normal.
- 100 to 125 mg/dL (5.6 to 6.9 mmol/L) is diagnosed as prediabetes.
- 126 mg/dL (7 mmol/L) or higher on two separate tests is diagnosed as diabetes.

Oral glucose tolerance test. This test is less commonly used than the others, except during pregnancy. You'll need to fast overnight and then drink a sugary liquid at the doctor's office. Blood sugar levels are tested periodically for the next two hours. Results are interpreted as follows:

- Less than 140 mg/dL (7.8 mmol/L) is normal.
- 140 to 199 mg/dL (7.8 mmol/L and 11.0 mmol/L) is diagnosed as prediabetes.
- 200 mg/dL (11.1 mmol/L) or higher after two hours suggests diabetes.

Screening. The American Diabetes Association recommends routine screening with diagnostic tests for type 2 diabetes in all adults age 45 or older and in the following groups:

- People younger than 45 who are overweight or obese and have one or more risk factors associated with diabetes
- Women who have had gestational diabetes

- People who have been diagnosed with prediabetes
- Children who are overweight or obese and who have a family history of type 2 diabetes or other risk factors

After a diagnosis

If you are given a diabetes diagnosis, your doctor or healthcare provider may order further tests to differentiate between type 1 and type 2 diabetes, since the two illnesses often call for distinct forms of therapy.

At least twice a year, and if there are any medication modifications, your doctor will perform the A1C test. Your age and other variables may affect your target A1C targets. The American Diabetes Association advises an A1C level under 7% for the majority of persons.

Additionally, you will have routine diagnostic exams to check for comorbid diseases or diabetes-related complications.

Treatment

Management of type 2 diabetes includes:

- Healthy eating
- Regular exercise
- Weight loss
- Possibly, diabetes medication or insulin therapy

- Blood sugar monitoring

These steps will help keep your blood sugar level closer to normal, which can delay or prevent complications.

Healthy eating

Contrary to popular perception, there's no specific diabetes diet. However, it's important to center your diet around:

- A regular schedule for meals and healthy snacks
- Smaller portion sizes
- More high-fiber foods, such as fruits, non starchy vegetables and whole grains
- Fewer refined grains, starchy vegetables and sweets
- Modest servings of low-fat dairy, low-fat meats and fish
- Healthy cooking oils, such as olive oil or canola oil
- Fewer calories

- Your health care provider may recommend seeing a registered dietitian, who can help you:

- Identify healthy choices among your food preferences
- Plan well-balanced, nutritional meals
- Develop new habits and address barriers to changing habits

- Monitor carbohydrate intake to keep your blood sugar levels more stable

Physical activity

Exercise is essential for weight loss or maintaining a healthy weight. It also helps to regulate blood sugar levels. Consult your primary healthcare provider to make sure the exercises are appropriate for you before starting or changing your exercise regimen.

aerobic exercise Pick a favorite aerobic exercise, such as walking, running, biking, or swimming. Adults should aim for 150 or more weekly minutes of moderate aerobic exercise, or at least 30 minutes on most days. Children should do 60 minutes of moderate to vigorous aerobic exercise each day.

resistance exercise increases your ability for daily chores, balance, and strength. Resistance training includes weightlifting, yoga, and calisthenics.

Type 2 diabetic adults should aim to complete two to three bouts of resistance training per week. Kids should engage in activities that improve their flexibility and strength at least three days a week. Climbing playground equipment, sports, and resistance training are a few instances of this.

Try to continue moving. To help control blood sugar levels, extended periods of inactivity, such as working at a computer, may be broken up. Spend a few minutes standing up, moving about, or doing some light exercise every 30 minutes.

Weight loss

Weight loss is followed by improved control of blood pressure, cholesterol, triglycerides, and blood sugar. If you are overweight, these indications may start to get better after you drop as little as 5% of your body weight. However, as you lose more weight, the benefits to your health and disease management will become more apparent.

Your doctor or nutritionist can help you set reasonable weight reduction goals and encourage you to make the required lifestyle changes.

Monitoring your blood sugar

Your healthcare provider will advise you on how often to monitor your blood sugar level to make sure it remains within your target range. You may need to check it once daily, either before or after exercise, for example. If you use insulin, you may need to repeat this many times per day.

Monitoring is often done using a blood glucose meter, a little device that you may use at home to determine how much sugar is in a drop of your blood. For your medical team to see your measurements, you should record them.

A continuous glucose monitoring gadget electronically checks your blood sugar levels every few minutes using a sensor that is implanted under your skin. Alarms may be sent by the system when levels are abnormally high or low, and data may be sent to a mobile device, such as your phone.

Diabetes medications

Your doctor may recommend insulin treatment or diabetic drugs that assist in reducing insulin levels if you are unable to maintain your target blood sugar level with diet and exercise. The following are examples of type 2 diabetic medications.

Metformin (Fortamet, Glumetza, others) Your doctor may give diabetic drugs that reduce insulin levels or insulin treatment if you are unable to maintain your target blood sugar level with diet and exercise. The following are some drug therapies for type 2 diabetes.

Some people experience B-12 deficiency and may need to take supplements. Other possible side effects, which may improve over time, include:

- Nausea
- Abdominal pain
- Bloating

- Diarrhea

Sulfonylureas help your body secrete more insulin. Examples include glyburide (DiaBeta, Glynase), glipizide (Glucotrol) and glimepiride (Amaryl). Possible side effects include:

- Low blood sugar
- Weight gain

Glinides stimulate the pancreas to secrete more insulin. They're faster acting than sulfonylureas, and the duration of their effect in the body is shorter. Examples include repaglinide and nateglinide. Possible side effects include:

- Low blood sugar
- Weight gain

Thiazolidinediones make the body's tissues more sensitive to insulin. Examples include rosiglitazone (Avandia) and pioglitazone (Actos). Possible side effects include:

- Risk of congestive heart failure
- Risk of bladder cancer (pioglitazone)
- Risk of bone fractures
- High cholesterol (rosiglitazone)
- Weight gain

DPP-4 inhibitors help reduce blood sugar levels but tend to have a very modest effect. Examples include sitagliptin (Januvia), saxagliptin (Onglyza) and linagliptin (Tradjenta). Possible side effects include:

- Risk of pancreatitis
- Joint pain

GLP-1 receptor agonists are injectable medications that slow digestion and help lower blood sugar levels. Their use is often associated with weight loss, and some may reduce the risk of heart attack and stroke. Examples include exenatide (Byetta, Bydureon), liraglutide (Saxenda, Victoza) and semaglutide (Rybelsus, Ozempic). Possible side effects include:

- Risk of pancreatitis
- Nausea
- Vomiting
- Diarrhea

SGLT2 inhibitors affect the blood-filtering functions in your kidneys by inhibiting the return of glucose to the bloodstream. As a result, glucose is excreted in the urine. These drugs may reduce the risk of heart attack and stroke in people with a high risk of those conditions. Examples include canagliflozin (Invokana), dapagliflozin (Farxiga) and empagliflozin (Jardiance). Possible side effects include:

- Risk of amputation (canagliflozin)

- Risk of bone fractures (canagliflozin)
- Risk of gangrene
- Vaginal yeast infections
- Urinary tract infections
- Low blood pressure
- High cholesterol

Other medications your doctor might prescribe in addition to diabetes medications include blood pressure and cholesterol-lowering medications, as well as low-dose aspirin, to help prevent heart and blood vessel disease.

Insulin therapy

Certain type 2 diabetics need insulin treatment. Nowadays, if blood sugar objectives aren't achieved with lifestyle modifications and other drugs, insulin treatment may be administered sooner rather than later.

The time it takes to start working and how long it takes to have an impact varies across different forms of insulin. For instance, long-acting insulin is made to function all day or overnight to maintain stable blood sugar levels. During mealtimes, short-acting insulin may be used.
What sort of insulin is best for you and when to take it will be decided by your doctor. Depending on how steady your blood sugar levels are, your insulin type, dose, and schedule may fluctuate. Most insulin varieties are administered through injection.

High triglycerides, diabetic ketoacidosis, and low blood sugar (hypoglycemia) are possible side effects of insulin.

Weight-loss surgery

Your digestive system's structure and functionality are altered by weight-loss surgery. You might control type 2 diabetes, your weight, and other obesity-related diseases with the aid of this operation. There are several surgical methods, but they all work by reducing the amount of food you can consume. Additionally, certain operations restrict how much nutrition you may absorb.

Surgery for weight reduction is only one element of a comprehensive therapeutic strategy. Additionally, your treatment plan will include advice on your exercise routine, food, and nutritional supplements.

In general, persons with type 2 diabetes with a body mass index (BMI) of 35 or above may be candidates for weight-loss surgery. Using weight and height, the BMI formula calculates an estimate of body fat. Surgery may be a possibility for someone with a BMI under 35, depending on the severity of their diabetes or concomitant diseases.

Surgery for weight reduction requires a lifetime commitment to behavioral adjustments. Osteoporosis and dietary deficits are long-term adverse effects.

Pregnancy

Women with type 2 diabetes will probably need to modify their treatment regimens and follow diets that strictly limit their carbohydrate consumption. Many pregnant women may need insulin therapy and may have to stop using other drugs or treatments, such as blood pressure meds.

Pregnancy increases the chance of having diabetic retinopathy or seeing the disease become worse. Visit an ophthalmologist throughout each trimester of your pregnancy, one year after giving birth, or as recommended if you are pregnant or planning a pregnancy.

Signs of trouble

It's crucial to regularly check your blood sugar levels to prevent serious consequences. Be mindful of the following indications and symptoms that may point to erratic blood sugar levels and the need for urgent attention:

High blood sugar (hyperglycemia). Eating certain foods or too much food, being sick, or not taking medications at the right time can cause high blood sugar. Signs and symptoms include:

- Frequent urination

- Increased thirst
- Dry mouth
- Blurred vision
- Fatigue
- Headache

Hyperglycemic Hyperosmolar nonketotic syndrome (HHNS). This life-threatening condition includes a blood sugar reading higher than 600 mg/dL (33.3 mmol/L). HHNS may be more likely if you have an infection, are not taking medicines as prescribed, or take certain steroids or drugs that cause frequent urination. Signs and symptoms include:

- Dry mouth
- Extreme thirst
- Drowsiness
- Confusion
- Dark urine
- Seizures

Diabetic ketoacidosis

Diabeticketoacidosis happens when the body starts using fat as fuel instead of sugar because of a lack of insulin. As a consequence, the bloodstream begins to accumulate acids known as ketones. Certain diseases, pregnancy, trauma, and drugs, including SGLT2 inhibitors for diabetes, may cause diabetic ketoacidosis.

Type 2 diabetes normally results in a milder form of diabetic ketoacidosis, although the acids' toxicity may be fatal. Ketoacidosis may cause: In addition to the signs and symptoms of hypoglycemia, such as increased thirst and frequent urination:

- Nausea
- Vomiting
- Abdominal pain
- Shortness of breath
- Fruity-smelling breath

Low blood sugar

Low blood sugar is referred to as when your blood sugar level falls below your desired range (hypoglycemia). Many things might cause your blood sugar to decrease, including missing meals, accidentally taking more medicine than normal, or engaging in more physical activity than usual. Some warning signs and symptoms are:

- Sweating
- Shakiness
- Weakness
- Hunger
- Irritability
- Dizziness
- Headache
- Blurred vision
- Heart palpitations

- Slurred speech
- Drowsiness
- Confusion

If you experience any of the warning signs or symptoms of low blood sugar, you should immediately consume fruit juice, glucose tablets, hard candies, or another source of sugar to fast boost your blood sugar level. In 15 minutes, repeat your blood test. Repeat the sugar consumption if the levels are not where you want them to be. After levels stabilize, have a meal.

You will need an emergency infusion of the hormone glucagon, which accelerates the release of sugar into the blood if you lose consciousness.

Chapter 10

Quick and Healthy Meals for People With Diabetes and how you can prevent Diabetes.

Any meal is OK if you have diabetes. The secret is to keep track of quantities, balance your diet, and consume about the same amount of carbs at each meal.

Along with recipes for breakfast, lunch, and supper, these four-pointers may get you going.

1. To find out how various meals impact your blood sugar levels, do a blood sugar test.
2. Limit the grams of carbohydrates you consume at each meal. This typically amounts to 45–75 grams three times each day..
3. In every meal, strike a balance between carbs, fiber, and protein. Using the plate approach makes this simple. Place vegetables on half of your plate, followed by a healthy carbohydrate like brown rice, black beans, or whole-wheat pasta, then a healthy protein like chicken breast, fish, lean beef, or tofu on the other half. Depending on how many carbs you want to consume at that meal, add a tiny piece of fruit and some low-fat or fat-free milk or yogurt.
4. Consume healthy fats from foods like nuts, avocados, seafood, olives, and other plants.

Avoid consuming saturated fats from dairy products such as cheese, butter, and beef.
If any of the recipes included below call for fewer carbohydrates per serving than your physician or healthcare team has advised, add additional carbs to the meal as a whole. This might be a tiny piece of whole-grain bread, fruit or vegetable, nonfat yogurt or milk, or both.

Prevention

Type 1 diabetes can't be prevented. But the healthy lifestyle choices that help treat prediabetes, type 2 diabetes and gestational diabetes can also help prevent them:

- Eat nutritious meals. Pick meals with more fiber and fewer calories and fat. Emphasize whole grains, veggies, and fruits. Eat a variety of foods to avoid becoming bored.
- Get moving more often. On most days of the week, try to engage in around 30 minutes of moderate aerobic exercise. Or try to do 150 minutes or more of moderate aerobic exercise each week. Take a brisk daily stroll as an example. Break up a lengthy exercise into shorter periods throughout the day if you are unable to fit it in.
  Lose any extra weight. If you are overweight, even a 7% weight loss may reduce your chance

of developing diabetes. If you weigh 200 pounds (90.7 kilograms), for instance, decreasing 14 pounds (6.4 kilograms) may reduce your chance of developing diabetes.

However, avoid attempting to reduce weight when pregnant. Find out from your doctor how much weight you may safely acquire while expecting.

Work on long-term improvements to your food and exercise routines to maintain a healthy weight. Keep in mind the advantages of decreasing weight, like a healthier heart, increased energy, and improved self-esteem.

Drugs are a possibility on occasion. Type 2 diabetes risk may be decreased by oral diabetic medications like metformin (Glumetza, Fortamet, and others). However, adopting a healthy lifestyle is crucial. Check your blood sugar at least once a year if you have prediabetes to ensure type 2 diabetes has not yet manifested.